Keto Slow Cooker Recipes for Daily Healthy Meals

A Collection of 50 Delicious Keto Recipes for Your Daily Meals

Katherine Lowe

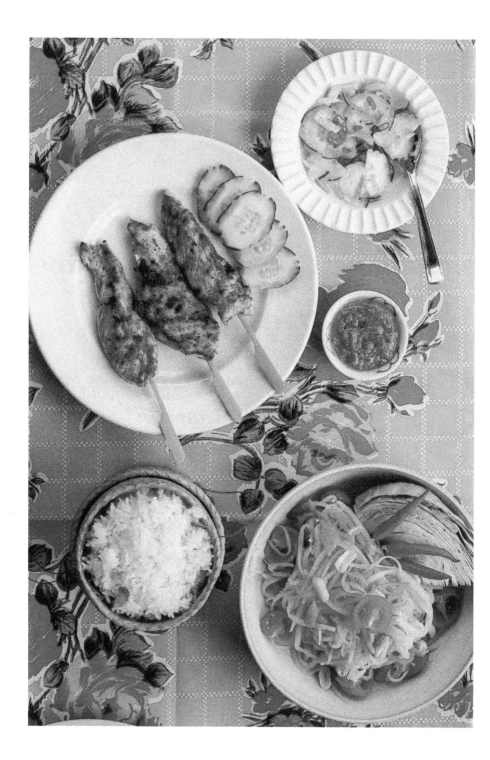

sources. Please consult a licensed professional before attempting any techniques outlined in this book.

By reading this document, the reader agrees that under no circumstances is the author responsible for any losses, direct or indirect, which are incurred as a result of the use of information contained within this document, including, but not limited to, — errors, omissions, or inaccuracies.

Table of Contents

Parsley Wine Tomato-Braised Tuna

Preparation time: 15 minutes

Cooking time: 2 hours & 30 minutes

Servings: 8

Ingredients:

- 2 tuna fillets (3 pounds)
- ½ cup olive oil
- 1 small red onion, chopped
- 6 garlic cloves, minced
- 3 cups gluten-free, sugar-free tomato sauce
- 1 cup dry white wine
- 6 tablespoons drained and rinsed capers
- 4 tablespoons chopped fresh parsley
- 2 bay leaves
- Sea salt
- Freshly ground black pepper

Directions:

1. Place the tuna in a bowl of cold salted water to soak for about 12 minutes. Drain well and pat dry using paper towels.

2. Place a skillet over a medium-high flame and heat 2 tablespoons of oil. Sauté the onion and garlic until the onion is translucent. Transfer into the slow cooker.

7

3. Stir the wine, tomato, marinara sauce, capers, bay leaves, and parsley into the slow cooker. Cover and cook within 1 hour on high.

4. Put the skillet over medium-high heat and heat the rest of the oil. Brown the tuna fillets all over, then place into the slow cooker. Cover and cook for 1 hour and 30 minutes on high, or until the tuna is cooked.

Nutrition:

- Calories: 155
- Fat: 16.5g
- Carbs: 8g
- Protein: 40g

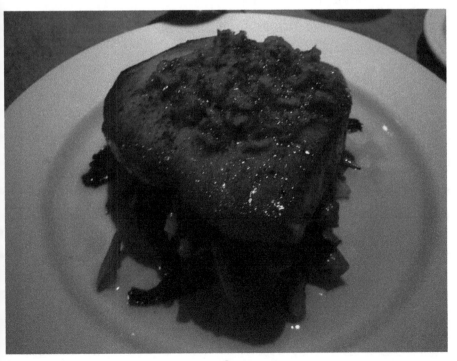

Garlic Cabbage Beef Soup

Preparation time : 15 minutes

Cooking time : 10 hours

Servings: 6

Ingredients:
- 2 tablespoons coconut oil
- 8 ounces beef stew meat, diced
- Kosher salt
- Freshly ground black pepper
- 8 ounces smoked beef sausage, diced
- 1 onion, finely chopped
- 3 cups shredded cabbage
- 2 cups beef broth
- 1 (15-ounce) can tomato sauce
- 2 garlic cloves, minced
- 2 bay leaves
- 3 tablespoons chopped fresh parsley
- 1 cup sour cream

Directions:

1. Warm-up coconut oil over medium-high heat in a large skillet. Generously season the meat with salt and pepper and add it to the skillet, along with the sausage.

2. Cook until the meat is browned on all sides, about 6 minutes. Transfer the beef and sausage to the slow cooker.

3. Move it back to the skillet to medium-high heat and add the onion. Sauté until softened, about 4 minutes. Transfer the onion to the slow cooker.

4. Add the cabbage, beef broth, tomato sauce, garlic, and bay leaves to the slow cooker. Cover and cook for 8 to 10 hours on low. Discard the bay leaves and serve hot, garnished with the parsley and a dollop of sour cream.

Nutrition:

- Calories: 329
- Fat: 26g
- Carbs: 9g
- Protein: 16g

Mushrooms & Bell Pepper Cheesesteak

Preparation time : 15 minutes

Cooking time: 8 hours

Servings: 6

Ingredients:

- 2 tablespoons coconut oil
- 1 onion, thinly sliced
- 8 ounces cremini or button mushrooms, sliced
- 1 green bell pepper, strips
- 1 red bell pepper, strips
- 1½ pounds rib-eye steak
- ¾ teaspoon kosher salt
- ¾ teaspoon freshly ground black pepper

Directions:

1. In a large skillet, warm up the coconut oil over medium-high heat. Sauté the onion until beginning to soften, about 3 minutes.

2. Put the mushrooms, then continue to sauté until the mushrooms begin to brown, about 5 minutes. Transfer the mixture to the slow cooker.

3. Put the green plus red bell peppers in the slow cooker and stir to mix. Return the skillet to medium-high heat. Flavor the steak with the salt and pepper and add it to the skillet.

4.   Cook until browned, within 2 minutes per side. Transfer the steak to the slow cooker, placing it on top of the vegetables. Cover and cook within 8 hours on low.

5.   Remove the steak from the cooker and let it rest for a couple of minutes. Leave the slow cooker on and keep it covered.

6.   Slice the steak into thin strips and return them to the slow cooker. Place the provolone cheese over the top, replace the cover, and let it sit for a few minutes until the cheese is melty. Serve hot.

Nutrition:

- Calories: 734
- Fat: 59g
- Carbs: 8g
- Protein: 43g

Lemon Garlic Shrimp Scampi

Preparation time: 15 minutes

Cooking time: 1 hour & 30 minutes

Servings: 6

Ingredients:

- 1 lb. raw shrimp, peeled and deveined
- Juice of one fresh lemon
- 1/2 cup chicken broth
- 3 minced garlic cloves
- 4 tbsp butter
- 2 tbsp fresh parsley
- Salt and pepper as desired

Directions:

1. Adjust the heat of the slow cooker to high. Combine the chicken broth, lemon juice, butter, garlic, parsley, salt, and pepper in the crockpot. Stir thoroughly. Put the shrimp in, mixing well. Cook within 1 hour and 30 minutes. Serve.

Nutrition:

- Calories: 250
- Fat: 13.7g
- Carb: 4.6g
- Protein: 27g

Curry Beef

Preparation time: 15 minutes

Cooking time: 8 hours

Servings: 6

Ingredients:

- 1 cup diced tomatoes
- 1 (14-ounce) can coconut milk
- 1/3 cup water
- ¼ cup coconut oil, melted
- ¼ cup tomato paste
- 1 onion, diced
- 6 garlic cloves, minced
- 3 tablespoons grated fresh ginger
- 2 tablespoons ground cumin
- 1 teaspoon paprika
- 1 teaspoon kosher salt
- ½ teaspoon ground turmeric
- ½ teaspoon ground cardamom
- ½ teaspoon ground cinnamon
- ½ teaspoon ground cloves
- ½ teaspoon cayenne pepper
- ¼ teaspoon ground nutmeg
- 1 (1½-pound) beef chuck roast, cut into ½-by-2-inch strips

- 1/3 cup chopped fresh cilantro

Directions:

1. In the slow cooker, stir the tomatoes, coconut milk, water, coconut oil, and tomato paste. Add the onion, garlic, ginger, cumin, paprika, salt, turmeric, cardamom, cinnamon, cloves, cayenne, and nutmeg.

2. Add the beef and toss to mix well. Cover and cook within 8 hours on low. Serve hot, garnished with the cilantro.

Nutrition:
- Calories: 547
- Fat: 46g
- Carbs: 12g
- Protein: 26g

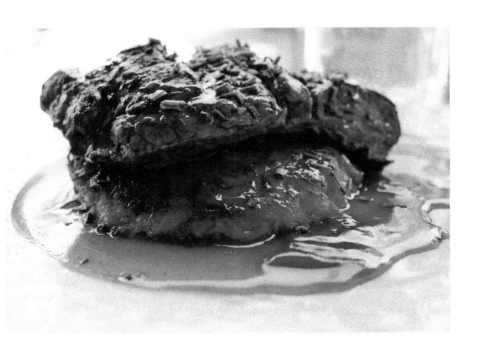

Heavy Creamy Herb Pork Chops

Preparation time: 15 minutes

Cooking time: 8 hours

Servings: 4

Ingredients:

- ¾ cup chicken or beef broth
- 2 tablespoons coconut oil, melted
- 1 tablespoon Dijon mustard
- 2 garlic cloves, minced
- 1 tablespoon paprika
- 1 tablespoon onion powder
- 1 teaspoon dried oregano
- 1 teaspoon dried basil
- 1 teaspoon dried parsley
- 1 onion, thinly sliced
- 4 thick-cut boneless pork chops
- 1 cup heavy (whipping) cream

Directions:

1. In the slow cooker, stir the broth, coconut oil, mustard, garlic, paprika, onion powder, oregano, basil, and parsley.

2. Add the onion and pork chops and toss to coat. Cover and cook within 8 hours on low or 4 hours on high. Transfer the chops to a serving platter.

3. Transfer the remaining juices and onion in the slow cooker to a blender, add the heavy cream, and process until smooth. Put the sauce over the pork chops, then serve hot.

Nutrition:
- Calories: 470
- Fat: 32g
- Carbs: 7g
- Protein: 39g

Mushroom Beef Stroganoff

Preparation time: 15 minutes

Cooking time: 8 hours

Servings : 6

Ingredients:

- 2 pounds beef stew meat, cut into 1-inch cubes
- 4 bacon slices, diced
- 8 ounces cremini or button mushrooms, quartered
- 1 onion, halved and sliced
- 2 garlic cloves, minced
- 1 cup beef broth
- ¼ cup tomato paste
- 1 teaspoon smoked paprika
- ½ teaspoon kosher salt
- ¼ teaspoon freshly ground black pepper
- 1½ cups sour cream
- 2 tablespoons minced fresh parsley

Directions:

1. In the slow cooker, stir the beef, bacon, mushrooms, onion, garlic, beef broth, tomato paste, paprika, salt, and pepper. Cover and cook within 8 hours on low. Stir in the sour cream, then serve hot, garnished with the parsley.

Nutrition:

- Calories: 594
- Fat: 47g
- Carb: 7g
- Protein: 35g

Ginger Cream Sauce Pork Loin

Preparation time: 15 minutes

Cooking time: 8 hours

Servings: 6

Ingredients:

For the pork:

- 1 tablespoon erythritol
- 2 teaspoons kosher salt
- 1 teaspoon garlic powder
- 1 teaspoon ground ginger
- ½ teaspoon ground cinnamon
- ½ teaspoon ground cloves
- ½ teaspoon red pepper flakes
- ¼ teaspoon freshly ground black pepper
- 1 (2-pound) pork shoulder roast
- ½ cup of water

For the sauce:

- 2 tablespoons unsalted butter
- 3 tablespoons minced fresh ginger
- 2 shallots, minced
- 1 tablespoon minced garlic
- 2/3 cup dry white wine
- 1 cup heavy (whipping) cream

Directions:

1. In a small bowl, stir the erythritol, salt, garlic powder, ginger, cinnamon, cloves, red pepper flakes, and black pepper. Rub the seasoning mixture all over the pork and place it in the slow cooker.

2. Pour the water into the cooker around the pork. Cover and cook within 8 hours on low. Remove, then let it rest for about 5 minutes.

3. While the pork rests, melt the butter in a small saucepan over medium heat. Stir in the ginger, shallots, and garlic.

4. Add the white wine and bring to a boil. Cook, stirring, until the liquid is reduced to about ¼ cup, about 5 minutes.

5. Mix in the heavy cream, then continue to boil, stirring until the sauce thickens, 3 to 5 minutes more. Slice the pork and serve it with the sauce spooned over the top.

Nutrition:

- Calories: 488
- Fat: 40g
- Carb: 5g
- Protein: 27g

Toasted Almond Braised Beef

Preparation time: 15 minutes

Cooking time: 9 hours

Servings: 6

Ingredients:

- ¼ cup of coconut oil
- 1 medium onion, diced
- 2 teaspoons ground cumin
- 1½ teaspoons kosher salt
- ½ teaspoon freshly ground black pepper
- ½ teaspoon ground cinnamon
- ½ teaspoon ground ginger
- 1 cup dry red wine
- 1 (1¼-pound) beef chuck roast, cut into 2-inch pieces
- Grated zest and juice of 1 orange
- 1 cup heavy (whipping) cream
- 5 tablespoons unsalted butter
- ½ cup ground toasted almonds
- ¼ cup chopped fresh cilantro

Directions:

1. In a large skillet, warm-up coconut oil over medium-high heat. Add the onion and sauté until soft, about 5 minutes. Add the cumin, salt, pepper, cinnamon, and ginger. Sauté for 1 minute more.

2. Mix in the red wine, then boil within 1 to 2 minutes, scraping up any browned bits from the pan's bottom. Transfer the mixture to the slow cooker.

3. Stir in the beef, orange zest, and orange juice. Cover and cook for 9 hours on low or 4½ hours on high.

4. Stir in the heavy cream plus butter until the butter melts, and both are well incorporated. Serve hot, garnished with the almonds and cilantro.

Nutrition:

- Calories: 747
- Fat: 56g
- Carbs: 9g
- Protein: 47g

Coconut Pumpkin Pork Stew

Preparation time: 15 minutes

Cooking time: 8 hours

Servings: 8

Ingredients:

- 2 tablespoons coconut oil
- 1½ pounds boneless pork ribs
- Kosher salt
- Freshly ground black pepper
- ½ onion, chopped
- 1 garlic clove, minced
- 1 jalapeño pepper, seeded and minced
- 1 teaspoon minced fresh ginger
- 1½ cups chicken broth
- 3 cups canned coconut milk
- 1 cup pumpkin purée
- ¼ cup all-natural peanut butter
- ¼ cup erythritol
- 1 teaspoon freshly squeezed lime juice
- ¼ cup chopped fresh cilantro
- ½ cup chopped toasted peanuts

Directions:

1. In a large skillet, heat-up coconut oil over medium-high heat. Flavor the pork with salt and pepper and add it to the skillet. Cook until browned on both sides, about 6 minutes. Transfer to the slow cooker.

2. Return the skillet to medium-high heat and add the onion, garlic, jalapeño, and ginger. Sauté until the onions are softened, about 3 minutes. Mix in the chicken broth and boil within 1 minute.

3. Stir in the coconut milk, pumpkin, peanut butter, and erythritol until smooth. Pour the mixture into the slow cooker. Cover and cook for 8 hours on low.

4. Remove the meat from the slow cooker, cut it into bite-size pieces, or shred it using two forks. Return the meat to the cooker. Stir in the lime juice. Serve hot, garnished with the cilantro and peanuts.

Nutrition:

- Calories: 492
- Fat: 41g
- Carb: 11g
- Protein: 24g

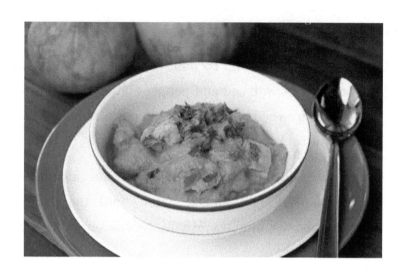

Ginger Spinach Chicken

Preparation time: 15 minutes

Cooking time: 5 hours

Servings: 8

Ingredients:

- 1/2 cup liquid aminos
- 1 tbsp fresh ginger, minced
- 8 chicken thighs
- 2 cups of water
- 1 tbsp garlic powder
- 1 tsp blackstrap molasses
- Salt and pepper to taste
- 2 cups spinach, whole leaves

Directions:

1. Mix the water and liquid aminos. Put this mixture in the crockpot. Add all the other spices and mix this in thoroughly as well.

2. Place the chicken thighs in the liquid in the slow cooker. Adjust the heat setting to high heat and put the lid on. Cook for 5 hours.

3. Add the spinach to the mixture in the crockpot. Recover and cook on high for ten minutes, stirring occasionally. Serve hot.

Nutrition:

- Calories: 472
- Fat: 35.7g
- Carb:3.8g
- Protein: 32.7g

Ghee Salmon with Fresh Cucumber Salad

Preparation time: 15 minutes

Cooking time: 3 hours

Servings: 8

Ingredients:

- 4 x 4oz Wild salmon fillets
- 2 tsp Tandoori spice
- 1 tsp salt
- 1 tsp black pepper
- 4 tbsp ghee
- Cucumber Salad
- 1 English cucumber
- 1 cup arugula
- ½ cup parsley
- ¼ cup lemon juice
- 2 tbsp extra virgin olive oil

Directions:

1. Heat-up ghee in a skillet over medium heat along with tandoori spice for a minute. Place salmon fillets in the slow cooker, skin side down, sprinkle with salt, black pepper, and pour Tandoori butter over salmon.

2. Cook on high for 3.5 hours. While salmon is cooking, dice the cucumber, and toss with arugula, parsley, lemon juice, and extra virgin olive oil. Serve salmon with fresh cucumber salad.

Nutrition:

- Calories: 413
- Carbs: 4g
- Fat: 34g
- Protein: 25g

Short Ribs

Preparation time: 15 minutes

Cooking time: 4 hours

Servings: 8

Ingredients:

- 4lbs. short ribs, bone-in
- 8 peppercorns
- 2 cups low-sodium beef
- 1 onion, diced
- 2 carrots, peeled, diced
- 2 celery stalks, diced
- 4 cloves, minced
- 1 tsp thyme
- 1 tsp rosemary
- 2 bay leaves
- 2 tsp salt
- 2 tsp black pepper
- Extra virgin olive oil

Directions:

1. Heat-up 4 tbsp extra virgin olive oil in a skillet. Add onions and garlic, and sauté until brown. Place onion mixture in the slow cooker, add short ribs, carrots, celery stalk, cloves, thyme, rosemary, peppercorns, bay leaves, salt, and black pepper. Cook on high for 4 hours.

Nutrition:

- Calories: 520
- Fat: 24g
- Carbs: 3.7g
- Protein: 67g

Cilantro Chili Verde

Preparation time: 15 minutes

Cooking time: 7 hours

Servings: 8

Ingredients:

- 1½lbs. pork shoulder
- ½ lb. sirloin, cubed
- 4 Anaheim chilis, stemmed
- 6 minced garlic cloves
- ½ cup cilantro, chopped
- 2 onions, peeled and sliced
- 2 tomatoes, chopped.
- 1 tbsp tomato paste
- 1 lime
- 1 tbsp cumin
- 1 tbsp oregano
- Extra virgin olive oil

Directions:

1. Slice pork shoulder into 1" cubes, and set slow cooker to medium. Heat-up four tbsp extra virgin olive oil in a skillet, add onions, Anaheim chilies, garlic, and sauté for 2 minutes.

2. Place skillet mixture into the slow cooker, add pork shoulder, sirloin, and stir. Add tomatoes, cilantro, tomato paste, cumin, oregano, and salt to the pot. Cover and cook for 7 hours. Squeeze a little lime in each bowl when serving.

Nutrition:

- Calories: 262
- Fat: 16g
- Carbs: 6g
- Protein: 23g

Thai Zucchini Lasagna

Preparation Time: 45 minutes

Cooking Time: 4 hours

Servings: 8

Ingredients:

For the zoodles:

- 4 large zucchinis
- 1 tbsp salt

For the lasagna:

- 2 tbsp coconut oil
- 1-pound extra-lean ground turkey
- 1 cup onion, diced
- 1 tbsp + 2 tsp fresh garlic, minced
- 1/2 tbsp fresh ginger, minced
- Pepper
- 1 cup light coconut milk
- 1/4 cup natural creamy peanut butter
- 1/4 cup reduced-sodium soy sauce
- 2 tbsp coconut sugar
- 1 tbsp rice vinegar
- 1 tbsp fresh lime juice
- 1 tbsp fish sauce
- 1-2 tbsp sriracha
- 15oz. light ricotta cheese

- 1 large egg
- 1/2 cup cilantro, roughly chopped
- 2 cups Nappa cabbage, roughly chopped
- 1/2 cup water chestnuts, diced
- 8 ounces mozzarella cheese, grated
- 1 large red pepper, diced

For garnish:

- Cilantro, diced
- Green onion, diced
- Roasted peanuts, diced
- Bean sprouts, roughly chopped

Directions:

1. Warm-up oven to 350 degrees. Cut the zucchini into thin using a mandolin, about 1/8 inch thick. Lay them out flat onto cookie sheets and sprinkle with 1 tbsp salt.

2. Bake within 15-20 minutes. Warm-up coconut oil over medium-high heat in the large pan. Put in the ground turkey, onion, garlic, ginger, plus a pinch of pepper. Cook within 10-12 minutes.

3. Once cooked, put the coconut milk, peanut butter, soy sauce, coconut sugar, rice vinegar, lime juice, fish sauce, plus 1 tbsp of the sriracha. Boil within 3 minutes. Adjust the heat to medium and simmer within 2-4 minutes. Stir occasionally, so it doesn't burn, then set aside.

4. Once the zoodles are finished, transfer it to a long piece of paper towel, cover with a different piece of paper towel, and then press out excess moisture.

5. Repeat the process with a fresh layer of paper towel over the top, then set aside. Beat the ricotta cheese, egg, and another pinch of pepper in a medium bowl, using a fork. Set aside.

6. For layer, spray the bottom of a slow cooker using cooking spray. Put in half of the turkey batter. Layer it with half the zucchini noodles in a single layer, then half the ricotta batter. Spread out the ricotta to "seal" in the zoodles.

7. Put half the cilantro on, then half the cabbage plus half the water chestnuts, finally, with half the mozzarella cheese.

8. Repeat the layers, except only use half of the rest of the mozzarella cheese on top. Then, add the diced red pepper on top of the last layer of mozzarella.

9. Cover your slow cooker and cook on low within 4-5 hours, or until everything is melted and the sides of the lasagna are brown. Sprinkle on the remaining cheese and let stand, covered until melted. Sprinkle with all the garnishes and devour!

Nutrition:

- Calories: 275
- Carbs: 13g
- Fat: 13g
- Protein: 26g

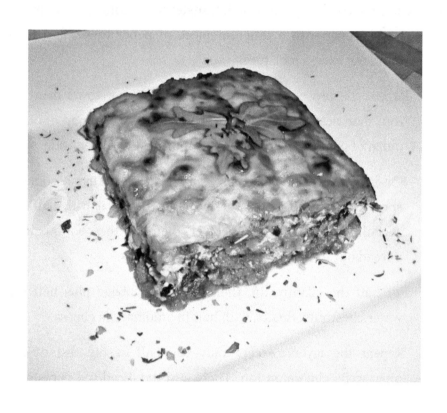

Keto Eggplants

Preparation Time: 15 minutes

Cooking Time: 7 hours

Servings: 14

Ingredients:

- 4 tbsps. olive oil
- 1 red onion
- 2 garlic cloves
- 1 lb. eggplant
- 7 ripe tomatoes
- 1 fennel bulb
- 4 sundried tomatoes
- 1 tsp. coriander seeds

Dressing:

- ¼ c. flat-leaf parsley
- ¼ c. basil
- 2 tsp. chives
- 2 tbsps. olive oil
- 1 juiced lemon

Topping:

- ½ c. toasted flaked almonds
- Keto bread for serving

Directions:

1. Peel the red onion and slice. Peel the garlic and crush it. Slice the bulb. Wash the tomatoes and cut. Wash parsley and chop, wash the basil leaves, chop the chives.

2. Squeeze the juice of a lemon. Open the crockpot, pour a little bit of olive oil into the crockpot, put the onions into the bottom, and add crushed garlic.

3. Slice the eggplant into thick slices and salt. Put them into the crockpot on top of the mix from onions and tomatoes, fennel, and sundried tomatoes.

4. Spread the coriander seeds, season well with salt and pepper. Cover and cook on low within 7 hours; the eggplant must be softened.

5. Prepare the dressing—mix parsley and basil, olive oil, juice of lemon, chives. Transfer the ready dish to a serving plate and drizzle with the dressing. Top with flaked almonds and serve with Keto bread.

Nutrition:

- Calories: 229
- Fat: 8.7g
- Protein: 31.7g
- Carbs: 4.7g

Italian Vegetable Bake

Preparation Time: 15 minutes

Cooking Time: 5 hours

Servings: 7

Ingredients:

- 3 garlic cloves
- 1 can tomato
- 1 bunch oregano
- ¼ tsp. chili flakes
- 11oz. baby aubergines
- 2 Courgettes
- ½ jar roasted red peppers
- 3 tomatoes
- 1 bunch basil
- Green salad

Directions:

1. Peel the garlic and mince. Chop tomatoes from the can. Wash the courgettes and slice, chop baby aubergines. Slice tomatoes. Open the crockpot, put the garlic, diced tomatoes, oregano leaves, chili, and some seasoning, add olive oil if necessary.

2. Add chopped aubergines, tomatoes, courgettes, red peppers, basil, and remaining oregano. Repeat vegetable layer, herb, and tomatoes. Push down well to compress, set on high for 5 hours. Serve with the basil leaves and the green salad.

Nutrition:
- Calories: 60
- Fat: 3.5g
- Protein: 2g
- Carbs: 6g

Spicy Maple Meatballs

Preparation Time: 15 minutes

Cooking Time: 5 hours

Servings: 11

Ingredients:

- 1 tbsp. olive oil
- ½ white onion
- 1 red bell pepper
- 1 green bell pepper
- 2 jalapeno peppers
- 1½ c. plain tomato sauce
- 1 c. maple syrup
- 2 tbsps. almond flour
- 2 tsp. ground allspice
- 1/8 tsp. liquid smoke
- 1 bag frozen vegan meatballs

Directions:

1. Peel the onion, chop it finely. Wash and slice peppers. Set aside. Add olive oil to the crockpot, add onion and peppers.

2. Take a medium bowl to add flour, maple syrup, tomato sauce, allspice, liquid smoke. Mix all until smooth consistency. Pour into the crockpot.

3. Add frozen meatballs. Cover and cook on low for 5 hours. The sauce should be thick and cover the meatballs. Serve warm over cauliflower rice.

Nutrition:

- Calories: 68
- Fat: 1.6g
- Protein: 7.2g
- Carbs: 6.6g

Spiced Cauliflower

Preparation Time: 10 minutes

Cooking Time: 2 hours

Servings: 13

Ingredients:

- 1 large cauliflower, cut into 1-inch pieces
- 1 medium onion, diced
- 1 medium tomato, dice
- 2 ginger roots, grate
- 2 garlic cloves
- 2 jalapeño peppers, sliced
- 1 tbsp cumin seeds
- ¼ tsp. cayenne pepper
- 1 tbsp. garam masala
- 1 tbsp. kosher salt
- 1 tsp. turmeric
- 3 tbsp. vegetable oil
- 1 tbsp. fresh cilantro, chop

Directions:

1. Put in the crockpot cauliflower florets, onion, tomato, ginger, garlic, peppers, masala, salt, turmeric, oil, and all the other fixing except fresh cilantro. Stir everything well. Cover and put on low for 2 hours. Serve with fresh cilantro.

Nutrition:

- Calories: 87
- Fat: 2.1g
- Protein: 10.3g
- Carbs: 7g

Garlic-Parmesan Asparagus

Preparation Time: 10 minutes

Cooking Time: 1 hour

Servings: 6

Ingredients:

- 2 tbsps. olive oil extra virgin
- 2 tsp. minced garlic
- 1 egg
- ½ tsp. garlic salt
- 12oz. fresh asparagus
- 1/3 cup of Parmesan cheese, shred
- pepper

Directions:

1. Take a medium-sized bowl combine oil, garlic, cracked egg, and salt. Whisk everything well. Cover the green beans and coat them well.

2. Spread the cooking spray over the crockpot's bottom, put the coated asparagus, season with the shredded cheese. Toss everything finely.

3. Cover and cook on high for 1 hour. Once the time is over, you may also season with the rest of the cheese.

Nutrition:

- Calories: 60
- Fat: 4.4g
- Protein: 2.2g
- Carbs: 4.7g

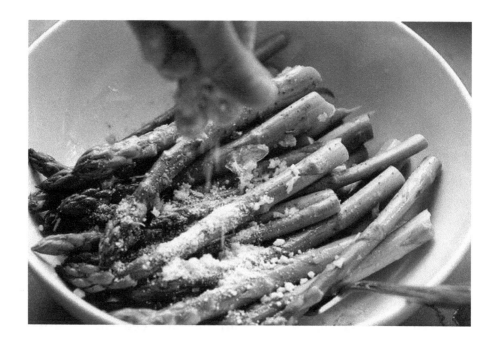

Spinach Artichoke Casserole

Preparation Time: 10 minutes

Cooking Time: 6 hours

Servings: 10

Ingredients:

- 8 large eggs
- 3/4 cup unsweetened almond milk
- 5 ounces fresh spinach chopped
- 6 ounces artichoke hearts chopped
- 1 cup grated parmesan
- 3 minced garlic cloves
- 1 tsp salt
- 1/2 tsp pepper
- 3/4 cup coconut flour
- 1 tbsp baking powder

Directions:

1. Oil the inside of a 6-quart slow cooker. In a large bowl, whisk the eggs, almond milk, spinach, artichoke hearts, 1/2 cup of the parmesan or nutritional yeast, garlic, salt, and pepper.

2. Add coconut flour and baking powder and whisk until very well combined. Spread mixture into the slow cooker and sprinkle remaining 1/2 cup parmesan over. Cook on high within 2 to 3

hours or low for 4 to 6 hours. Sprinkle with chopped fresh basil.

Nutrition:

- Calories: 141
- Fat: 7.1g
- Protein: 10g
- Carbs: 7.8g

French Onion Soup

Preparation Time: 10 minutes

Cooking Time: 4 hours

Servings: 8

Ingredients:

- 2 large white onions, sliced thin
- 6 cups low-sodium beef or bone broth
- 2 cups cheese, grated
- 1 tbsp ghee or butter
- 1 garlic clove, minced
- 1/2 tsp salt
- 1/2 tsp dried thyme
- 1/4 tsp pepper
- 1 bay leaf

Directions:

1. Add all the fixing except the cheese to the slow cooker. Stir to mix well. Cook high 3-4 hours, low 6-8. Remove bay leaf.

2. Preheat broiler. Ladle the soup evenly into bowls & top evenly with shredded cheese. Arrange bowls on a large baking sheet.

3. Place the baking sheet carefully under the broiler and broil a few minutes or until cheese is melted and slightly brown. Serve and enjoy!

Nutrition:

- Calories: 150
- Fat: 10.3g
- Protein: 10.4g
- Carbs: 4.2g

Vegan Rice and Beans

Preparation Time: 5 minutes

Cooking Time: 4 hours

Servings: 6

Ingredients:

- 2 packages frozen cauliflower rice (12oz each.)
- 2 cans black soybeans, drained
- 1/2 cup hulled hemp seeds
- 1 cup vegetable broth or stock
- 3 tbsp olive oil
- 2 tsp garlic powder
- 1 tsp onion powder
- 1 tsp cumin
- 1 tsp chili powder
- 1/2 tsp cayenne powder
- 1 tbsp Mexican oregano
- Garnishes of choice

Directions:

1. Add all the fixing except the Mexican oregano to the slow cooker, then mix around as best as possible. Let cook on High within 3-4 hours, until the "rice" is tender. Stir in oregano, then serve.

Nutrition:

- Calories: 299
- Fat: 20.2g
- Protein: 19.3g
- Carbs: 4.9g

Broccoli Parmesan Soup

Preparation Time: 10 minutes

Cooking Time: 2 hours

Servings: 12

Ingredients:

- 2 cups of water
- 2 cups of chicken broth
- 5 cups of fresh broccoli florets, chopped
- 8oz. softened cream cheese
- 1 cup whipping cream
- 1/2 cup Parmesan cheese
- 2 ½ cups shredded Cheddar cheese
- 2 tbsp of softened unsalted butter
- Dash of thyme
- Salt and pepper to taste

Directions:

1. In your slow cooker, put the butter, softened cream cheese, whipping cream, chicken broth, water, and mix well. Once thoroughly combined, add the parmesan cheese.

2. Put the chopped broccoli crowns, thyme. Cover and cook on low within 3 hours or medium-high for 80 minutes.

3. Then simply give the soup a good stir and then add the 2 1/2 cups of shredded cheddar cheese. Stir a few times, allowing the

cheddar cheese to melt completely. Add the salt and pepper to taste.

Nutrition:

- Calories: 230
- Fat: 20g
- Protein: 9.8g
- Carbs: 3.8g

Zucchini Pasta

Preparation time: 15 minutes

Cooking time: 1 hour

Servings: 4

Ingredients:

- 2 zucchinis
- 1 teaspoon dried oregano
- 1 teaspoon dried basil
- 2 tablespoons butter
- ¼ teaspoon salt
- 5 tablespoons water

Directions:

1. Peel the zucchini and spiralize it with a veggie spiralizer. Dissolve the butter and mix it with the dried oregano, dried basil, salt, and water.

2. Place the spiralized zucchini in the slow cooker and add the spice mixture. Close the lid and cook the meal for 1 hour on low. Let the cooked pasta cool slightly. Serve it!

Nutrition:

- Calories: 68
- Fat: 6g
- Carbs: 3.5g
- Protein: 1.3g

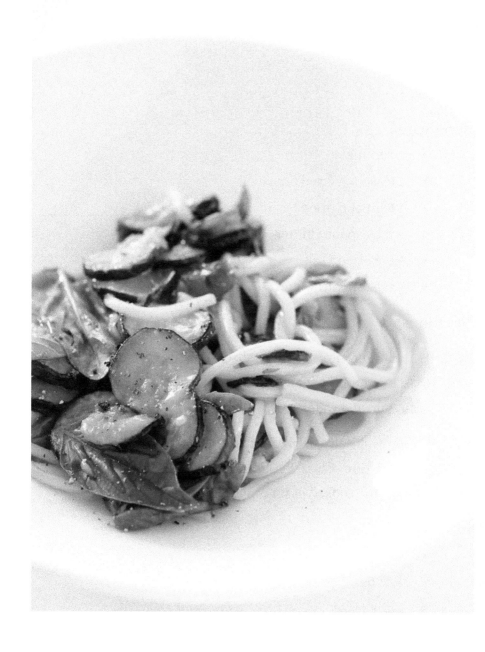

Chinese Broccoli

Preparation time: 15 minutes

Cooking time: 1 hour

Servings: 4

Ingredients:

- 1 tablespoon sesame seeds
- 1 tablespoon olive oil
- 10oz. broccoli
- 1 teaspoon chili flakes
- 1 tablespoon apple cider vinegar
- 3 tablespoons water
- ¼ teaspoon garlic powder

Directions:

1. Cut the broccoli into the florets and sprinkle with the olive oil, chili flakes, apple cider vinegar, and garlic powder.

2. Stir the broccoli and place it in the slow cooker. Add water and sesame seeds. Cook the broccoli for 1 hour on High. Transfer the cooked broccoli to serving plates and enjoy!

Nutrition:

- Calories: 69
- Fat: 4.9g
- Carbs: 5.4g
- Protein: 2.4g

Spaghetti Squash

Preparation time: 15 minutes

Cooking time: 4 hours

Servings: 5

Ingredients:

- 1-pound spaghetti squash
- 1 tablespoon butter
- ¼ cup of water
- 1 teaspoon ground black pepper
- ¼ teaspoon ground nutmeg

Directions:

1. Peel the spaghetti squash and sprinkle it with the ground black pepper and ground nutmeg. Pour water into the slow cooker.

2. Add butter and spaghetti squash. Close the lid and cook within 4 hours on low. Chop the spaghetti squash into small pieces and serve!

Nutrition:

- Calories: 50
- Fat: 2.9g
- Carbs: 0.1g
- Protein: 0.7g

Preparation time: 15 minutes

Mushroom Stew

Cooking time: 6 hours

Servings: 8

Ingredients:

- 10oz. white mushrooms, sliced
- 2 eggplants, chopped
- 1 onion, diced
- 1 garlic clove, diced
- 2 bell peppers, chopped
- 1 cup of water
- 1 tablespoon butter
- ½ teaspoon salt
- ½ teaspoon ground black pepper

Directions:

1. Place the sliced mushrooms, chopped eggplant, and diced onion into the slow cooker. Add the garlic clove and bell peppers.

2. Sprinkle the vegetables with salt and ground black pepper. Add butter and water and stir it gently with a wooden

spatula. Close the lid and cook the stew for 6 hours on low. Stir the cooked stew one more time and serve!

Nutrition:

- Calories: 71
- Fat: 1.9g
- Carbs: 13g
- Protein: 3g

Cabbage Steaks

Preparation time: 15 minutes

Cooking time: 2 hours

Servings: 4

Ingredients:

- 10oz. white cabbage
- 1 tablespoon butter
- ½ teaspoon cayenne pepper
- ½ teaspoon chili flakes
- 4 tablespoons water

Directions:

1. Slice the cabbage into medium steaks and rub them with the cayenne pepper and chili flakes. Rub the cabbage steaks with butter on each side.

2. Place them in the slow cooker and sprinkle with water. Close the lid and cook the cabbage steaks for 2 hours on High.

3. When the cabbage steaks are cooked, they should be tender to the touch. Serve the cabbage steak after 10 minutes of chilling.

Nutrition:

- Calories: 44
- Fat: 3g
- Carbs: 4.3g
- Protein: 1g

Mashed Cauliflower

Preparation time: 20 minutes

Cooking time: 3 hours

Servings: 5

Ingredients:

- 3 tablespoons butter
- 1-pound cauliflower
- 1 tablespoon full-fat cream
- 1 teaspoon salt
- 1 teaspoon ground black pepper
- 1oz. dill, chopped

Directions:

1. Wash the cauliflower and chop it. Place the chopped cauliflower in the slow cooker. Add butter and full-fat cream.

2. Add salt and ground black pepper. Stir the mixture and close the lid. Cook the cauliflower for 3 hours on High.

3. When the cauliflower is cooked, transfer it to a blender and blend until smooth. Place the smooth cauliflower in a bowl and mix it with the chopped dill. Stir it well and serve!

Nutrition:

- Calories: 101
- Fat: 7.4g
- Carbs: 8.3g
- Protein: 3.1g

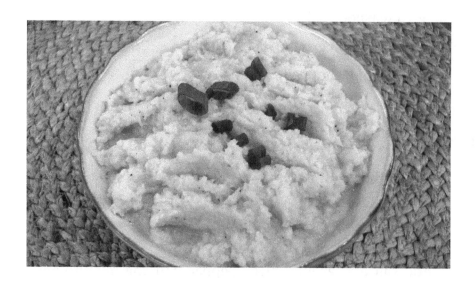

Bacon-Wrapped Cauliflower

Preparation time: 15 minutes

Cooking time: 7 hours

Servings: 4

Ingredients:

- 11oz. cauliflower head
- 3oz. bacon, sliced
- 1 teaspoon salt
- 1 teaspoon cayenne pepper
- 1oz. butter, softened
- ¾ cup of water

Directions:

1. Sprinkle the cauliflower head with the salt and cayenne pepper, then rub with butter. Wrap the cauliflower head in the sliced bacon and secure with toothpicks.

2. Put water into your slow cooker, then add the wrapped cauliflower head. Cook the cauliflower head for 7 hours on low. Then let the cooked cauliflower head cool for 10 minutes. Serve it!

Nutrition:

- Calories: 187
- Fat: 14.8g
- Carbs: 4.7g
- Protein: 9.5g

Cauliflower Casserole

Preparation time: 15 minutes

Cooking time: 7 hours

Servings: 5

Ingredients:

- 2 tomatoes, chopped
- 11oz. cauliflower chopped
- 5oz. broccoli, chopped
- 1 cup of water
- 1 teaspoon salt
- 1 tablespoon butter
- 5oz. white mushrooms, chopped
- 1 teaspoon chili flakes

Directions:

1. Mix the water, salt, and chili flakes. Place the butter in the slow cooker. Add a layer of the chopped cauliflower. Add the layer of broccoli and tomatoes. Add the mushrooms and pat down the mix to flatten.

2. Add the water and close the lid. Cook the casserole for 7 hours on low. Cool the casserole to room temperature and serve!

Nutrition:

- Calories: 61
- Fat: 2.6g
- Carbs: 8.1g
- Protein: 3.4g

Cauliflower Rice

Preparation time: 15 minutes

Cooking time: 2 hours

Servings: 5

Ingredients:

- 1-pound cauliflower
- 1 teaspoon salt
- 1 tablespoon turmeric
- 1 tablespoon butter
- ¾ cup of water

Directions:

1. Chop the cauliflower into tiny pieces to make cauliflower rice. You can also pulse in a food processor to get very fine grains of 'rice'

2. Place the cauliflower rice in the slow cooker. Add salt, turmeric, and water. Stir gently and close the lid. Cook the cauliflower rice for 2 hours on High. Strain the cauliflower rice and transfer it to a bowl. Add butter and stir gently. Serve it!

Nutrition:

- Calories: 48
- Fat: 2.5
- Carbs: 5.7
- Protein: 1.9

Curry Cauliflower

Preparation time: 15 minutes

Cooking time: 5 hours

Servings: 2

Ingredients:

- 10oz. cauliflower
- 1 teaspoon curry paste
- 1 teaspoon curry powder
- ½ teaspoon dried cilantro
- 1oz. butter
- ¾ cup of water
- ¼ cup chicken stock

Directions:

1. Chop the cauliflower roughly and sprinkle it with the curry powder and dried cilantro. Place the chopped cauliflower in the slow cooker. Mix the curry paste with the water. Add chicken stock and transfer the liquid to the slow cooker.

76

2.   Add butter and close the lid. Cook the cauliflower for 5 hours on low. Strain ½ of the liquid off and discard. Transfer the cauliflower to serving bowls. Serve it!

Nutrition:

- Calories: 158
- Fat: 13.3g
- Carbs: 8.9g
- Protein: 3.3g

Garlic Cauliflower Steaks

Preparation time: 15 minutes

Cooking time: 3 hours

Servings: 4

Ingredients:

- 14oz. cauliflower head
- 1 teaspoon minced garlic
- 4 tablespoons butter
- 4 tablespoons water
- 1 teaspoon paprika

Directions:

1. Wash the cauliflower head carefully and slice it into the medium steaks. Mix up the butter, minced garlic, and paprika.

2. Rub the cauliflower steaks with the butter mixture. Pour the water into the slow cooker. Add the cauliflower steaks and close the lid.

3. Cook the vegetables for 3 hours on High. Transfer the cooked cauliflower steaks to a platter and serve them immediately!

Nutrition:

- Calories: 129
- Fat: 11.7g
- Carbs: 5.8g
- Protein: 2.2g

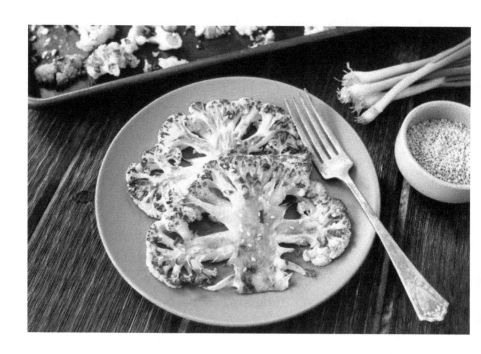

Zucchini Gratin

Preparation time: 10 minutes

Cooking time: 5 hours

Servings: 3

Ingredients:

- 1 zucchini, sliced
- 3oz. Parmesan, grated
- 1 teaspoon ground black pepper
- 1 tablespoon butter
- ½ cup almond milk

Directions:

1. Sprinkle the sliced zucchini with the ground black pepper. Chop the butter and place it in the slow cooker.

2. Transfer the sliced zucchini to the slow cooker to make the bottom layer. Add the almond milk. Sprinkle the zucchini with the grated cheese and close the lid.

3. Cook the gratin for 5 hours on low. Then let the gratin cool until room temperature. Serve it!

Nutrition:

- Calories: 229
- Fat: 19.6g
- Carbs: 5.9g
- Protein: 10.9g

Eggplant Gratin

Preparation time: 15 minutes

Cooking time: 5 hours

Servings: 7

Ingredients:

- 1 tablespoon butter
- 1 teaspoon minced garlic
- 2 eggplants, chopped
- 1 teaspoon salt
- 1 tablespoon dried parsley
- 4oz. Parmesan, grated
- 4 tablespoons water
- 1 teaspoon chili flakes

Directions:

1. Mix the dried parsley, chili flakes, and salt. Sprinkle the chopped eggplants with the spice mixture and stir well.

2. Place the eggplants in the slow cooker. Add the water and minced garlic. Add the butter and sprinkle with the grated parmesan.

3. Close the lid and cook the gratin for 5 hours on low. Open the lid and cool the gratin for 10 minutes. Serve it.

Nutrition:

- Calories: 107
- Fat: 5.4g
- Carbs: 10g
- Protein: 6.8g

Moroccan Eggplant Mash

Preparation time: 15 minutes

Cooking time: 7 hours

Servings: 4

Ingredients:

- 1 eggplant, peeled
- 1 jalapeno pepper
- 1 teaspoon curry powder
- ½ teaspoon salt
- 1 teaspoon paprika
- ¾ teaspoon ground nutmeg
- 2 tablespoons butter
- ¾ cup almond milk
- 1 teaspoon dried dill

Directions:

1. Chop the eggplant into small pieces. Place the eggplant in the slow cooker. Chop the jalapeno pepper and combine it with the eggplant.

2. Then sprinkle the vegetables with the curry powder, salt, paprika, ground nutmeg, and dried dill. Add almond milk and butter.

3. Close the lid and cook the vegetables for 7 hours on low. Cool the vegetables and then blend them until smooth with a hand blender. Transfer the cooked eggplant mash into the bowls and serve!

Nutrition:

- Calories: 190
- Fat: 17g
- Carbs: 10g
- Protein: 2.5g

Sautéed Bell Peppers

Preparation time: 15 minutes

Cooking time: 5 hours

Servings: 6

Ingredients:

- 8oz. bell peppers
- 7oz. cauliflower, chopped
- 2oz. bacon, chopped
- 1 teaspoon salt
- 1 teaspoon ground black pepper
- ¾ cup coconut milk, unsweetened
- 1 teaspoon butter
- 1 teaspoon thyme
- 1 onion, diced
- 1 teaspoon turmeric

Directions:

1. Discard the seeds from the bell peppers and chop them roughly. Place the bell peppers, cauliflower, and bacon in the slow cooker.

2.   Add the salt, ground black pepper, coconut milk, butter, milk, and thyme. Stir well, then add the diced onion. Add the turmeric and stir the mixture.

3.   Close the lid and cook 5 hours on low. When the meal is cooked, let it chill for 10 minutes and serve it!

Nutrition:
- Calories: 195
- Fat: 12.2g
- Carbs: 13.1g
- Protein: 6.7g

Simple Cashew Spread

Preparation time: 15 minutes

Cooking time: 6 hours

Servings: 4

Ingredients:

- 5 tbsps. cashews
- 1 tsp. apple cider vinegar
- 1 c. veggie stock
- 1 tbsp. Water

Directions:

1. In your Slow cooker, mix cashews and stock, stir, cover, and cook on low for 6 hours. Drain, transfer to your food processor, add vinegar and water, pulse well, divide into bowls, and serve as a party spread. Enjoy!

Nutrition:

- Calories: 221
- Fat: 6g
- Carbs: 9g

- Protein: 3g

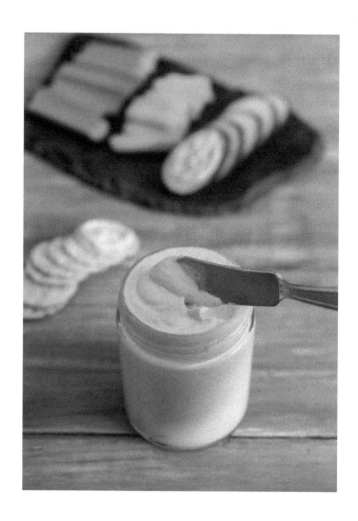

Beef Party Rolls

Preparation time: 15 minutes

Cooking time: 8 hours

Servings: 4

Ingredients:

- ½ lb. minced beef
- 1 green cabbage head
- ½ cup of chopped onion
- 1 cup of cauliflower rice
- 2oz. chopped white mushrooms
- ¼ cup of toasted pine nuts
- ¼ cup of raisins
- 2 minced garlic cloves
- 2 tbsps. chopped dill
- 1 tbsp. olive oil
- 25oz. tomato sauce
- Salt
- Black pepper
- ¼ cup of water

Directions:

1. In a bowl, mix beef with onion, cauliflower, mushrooms, pine nuts, raisins, garlic, dill, salt, and pepper and stir. Arrange cabbage leaves on a working surface, divide beef mix and wrap them well.

2. Add sauce and water to your Slow cooker, stir, add cabbage rolls, cover, and cook on low for 8 hours. Arrange rolls on a platter and serve as an appetizer with some of the pot drizzled sauce all over. Enjoy!

Nutrition:

- Calories: 361
- Fat: 6g
- Carbs: 12g
- Protein: 3g

Eggplant and Tomato Salsa

Preparation time: 15 minutes

Cooking time: 7 hours

Servings: 4

Ingredients:

- 1 ½ cup of chopped tomatoes
- 3 cups of cubed eggplant
- 2 tsp. capers
- 6oz. sliced green olives
- 4 minced garlic cloves
- 2 tsp. balsamic vinegar
- 1 tbsp. chopped basil
- Salt
- Black pepper

Directions:

1. In your Slow cooker, mix tomatoes with eggplant, capers, green olives, garlic, vinegar, basil, salt and pepper, toss, cover, and cook on low for 7 hours. Divide salsa into small bowls and serve as an appetizer. Enjoy!

Nutrition:

- Calories: 200
- Fat: 6g
- Carbs: 9g
- Protein: 2g

Carrots and Cauliflower Spread

Preparation time: 15 minutes

Cooking time: 7 hours

Servings: 4

Ingredients:

- 1 cup of sliced carrots
- 1½ cup of cauliflower florets
- 1/3 cup of cashews
- ½ cup of chopped turnips
- 2½ cups of water
- 1 cup of coconut milk
- 1 tsp garlic powder
- ¼ cup of nutritional yeast
- ¼ tsp smoked paprika
- ¼ tsp. mustard powder
- Salt
- Black pepper

Directions:

1. In your slow cooker, mix carrots with cauliflower, cashews, turnips, water, stir, cover, and cook on low for 7 hours.

2. Drain, transfer to a blender, add milk, garlic powder, yeast, paprika, mustard powder, salt, and pepper, blend well, divide into bowls and serve as a party spread. Enjoy!

Nutrition:

- Calories: 291
- Fat: 7g
- Carbs: 14g
- Protein: 3g

Mixed Veggies Spread

Preparation time: 15 minutes

Cooking time: 5 hours

Servings: 7

Ingredients:

- ½ riced cauliflower head
- 54oz. crushed tomatoes
- 10oz. chopped white mushrooms
- 2 cups of shredded carrots
- 2 cups of cubed eggplant
- 6 minced garlic cloves
- 2 tbsps. agave nectar
- 2 tbsps. balsamic vinegar
- 2 tbsps. tomato paste
- 1 tbsp. chopped basil
- 1 ½ tbsps. chopped oregano
- 1 ½ tsp. dried rosemary
- Salt
- Black pepper

Directions:

1. In your slow cooker, mix cauliflower with tomatoes, mushrooms, carrots, eggplant, garlic, agave nectar, vinegar, tomato paste, rosemary, salt, and pepper, stir, cover and cook on High for 5 hours.

2. Add basil and oregano, stir again, blend a bit using an immersion blender, divide into bowls and serve as a spread. Enjoy!

Nutrition:

- Calories: 301
- Fat: 7g
- Carbs: 10g
- Protein: 6g

Cashew Hummus

Preparation time: 15 minutes

Cooking time: 3 hours

Servings: 4

Ingredients:

- 1 cup of water
- 1 cup of cashews
- 2 tbsp tahini paste
- ¼ tsp garlic powder
- ¼ tsp onion powder
- ¼ cup of nutritional yeast
- Salt
- Black pepper
- ¼ tsp. mustard powder
- 1 tsp. apple cider vinegar

Directions:

1. In your slow cooker, mix water with cashews, yeast, salt, and pepper, stir, cover, and cook on High for 3 hours.

2. Transfer to your blender, add tahini, garlic powder, onion powder, mustard powder, and vinegar, pulse well, divide into bowls and serve. Enjoy!

Nutrition:

- Calories: 192
- Fat: 7g
- Carbs: 12g
- Protein: 4g

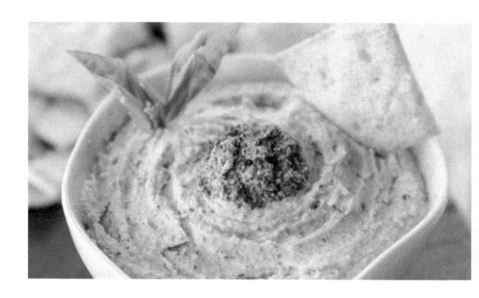

Bell Peppers Appetizer

Preparation time: 15 minutes

Cooking time: 4 hours

Servings: 5

Ingredients:

- 1 chopped yellow onion
- 2 tsp. olive oil
- 2 chopped celery ribs
- 1 tbsp. chili powder
- 3 minced garlic cloves
- 2 tsp. ground cumin
- 1½ tsp dried oregano
- 2½ cup of cauliflower rice
- 1 chopped tomato
- 1 chipotle pepper
- Salt
- Black pepper
- 5 colored bell peppers
- ½ cup of tomato sauce

Directions:

1. Heat-up pan with the oil over medium-high heat, add onion and celery, stir and cook for 5 minutes.

2. Add garlic, chili, cumin, oregano, cauliflower, tomato, chipotle, salt and pepper, stir, cook for a couple of minutes more, take off the heat, and stuff peppers with this mix.

3. Arrange bell peppers in your slow cooker, spread tomato sauce over them, cover, cook on low for 4 hours, arrange on a platter and serve them as appetizers. Enjoy!

Nutrition:

- Calories: 221
- Fat: 5g
- Carbs: 9g
- Protein: 3g

Artichoke and Coconut Spread

Preparation time: 15 minutes

Cooking time: 2 hours

Servings: 8

Ingredients:

- 28oz. chopped artichokes
- 10oz. spinach
- 8oz. coconut cream
- 1 chopped yellow onion
- 2 minced garlic cloves
- ¾ cup of coconut milk
- ½ cup of crumbled feta cheese
- 1/3 cup of mayonnaise
- 1 tbsp. red vinegar
- Salt
- Black pepper

Directions:

1. In your slow cooker, mix artichokes with spinach, coconut cream, onion, garlic, coconut milk, cheese, mayo, vinegar,

salt, and pepper, stir well, cover, and cook on low for 2 hours. Whisk spread well, divide into bowls and serve as an appetizer. Enjoy!

Nutrition:

- Calories: 305
- Fat: 14g
- Carbs: 9g
- Protein: 13g

Mushroom and Bell Peppers Spread

Preparation time: 15 minutes

Cooking time: 4 hours

Servings: 6

Ingredients:

- 2 c. chopped green bell peppers
- 1 c. chopped yellow onion
- 3 minced garlic cloves
- 1lb. chopped mushrooms
- 28oz. tomato sauce
- Salt
- Black pepper

Directions:

1. In your Slow cooker, mix bell peppers with onion, garlic, mushrooms, tomato sauce, salt and pepper, stir. Cook for 4 hours on low. Divide into bowls and serve as a spread. Enjoy!

Nutrition:

- Calories: 205
- Fat: 4g
- Carbs: 9g
- Protein: 3g

Lemon Perch

Preparation time: 5 minutes

Cooking time: 3 hours

Servings: 4

Ingredients:

- 1 slice of perch fillet
- 1 tablespoon of oil
- 1 tablespoon of salted butter
- ½ lemon juice
- 1 tablespoon of coconut flour
- 1 pinch of dill

Directions:

1. Cut the fillets into small pieces and roll in the flour. Sprinkle the juice of the half lemon in a bowl and combine the juice with a spoon of oil

2. Add salt to taste and mix the dill or any other aroma that you wish. Remove the excess flour from the fish and pour the emulsion onto the fish and make sure that all sides are covered

3. If you have a grill, put it on the Slow Cooker's bottom to get a steam cooking effect. Place a sheet of baking paper on the bottom of the Slow Cooker (or rest on the grid). Place the perch over the oven paper and cook for 3 hours on low, then serve.

Nutrition:

- Calories: 391
- Fat: 21.94g
- Carbs: 8.26g
- Protein 22.3g

Feta Black Olive Calamari

Preparation time: 15 minutes

Cooking time: 4 hours

Servings: 4

Ingredients:

- ½ cup of clean calamari
- 4 tablespoons of Greek feta
- 1 clove of garlic
- 28g of black olives
- 2 tablespoons of ghee
- 28g of peeled tomatoes
- 2 tablespoons of olive oil
- 1 pinch of salt
- 1 pinch of oregano

Directions:

1. Peel and mince the garlic. Cut the feta in cubes of about one centimeter. Fill the calamari heads with the feta cubes, some fresh parsley, and black olives.

2. Smear the calamari with the ghee using your hands. Soak the garlic in olive oil. Add the calamari and garlic sauce to a pan and sauté them for a couple of minutes.

3. Pour the oil used for the sauté on the bottom of the Slow Cooker, add the calamari, peeled tomatoes, oregano, salt, and pepper. Switch on the Slow Cooker setting it on high temperature, and let it cook for 4 hours.

Nutrition:

- Calories: 861
- Fat: 65.9g
- Carbs: 4.6
- Protein 39g

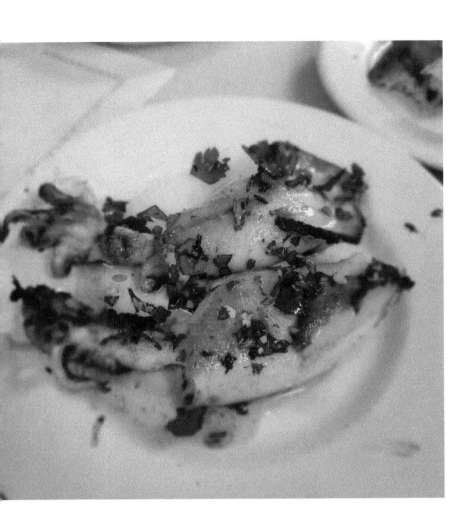

Lightning Source UK Ltd.
Milton Keynes UK
UKHW020755131222
413846UK00001B/9